Throw Out the Diet and Start Programming

By

Helen Hillyndale

I0424958

©Copyright 2019 Helen Hillyndale

A "diet" is described in the Oxford dictionary as "a limited range or amount of food, eaten in order to lose weight." Most people see a "diet" as the answer to their weight problems, never realizing that many of these "diets" are actually intended to be used to lose weight in the short term. The problem is that once they have reached their intended weight goal and ended the "diet", many people will inevitably revert to their old eating habits and begin to increase their weight until, in the majority of cases, they actually weigh more than they did when they first embarked on the "diet".

A "program" is described in the Oxford dictionary as "a plan of future events or things to be done" and also "to make something behave in a particular way". Programming for weight control is therefore a plan to control your weight in the long-term.

The purpose of this booklet is to help strengthen your resolve and make it possible to achieve your weight goals **permanently** and also help you avoid the pitfalls that can lead to you not achieving and maintaining your intended permanent weight loss. It doesn't contain a fixed weight loss program or diet but merely suggests the basics that such a program should contain. Above all it is an attempt to provide you with encouragement and knowledge of how to achieve a successful and permanent weight reduction. By following the suggestions in this booklet, your chances of achieving your permanent weight reduction goals can be greatly improved.

If you want to lose weight permanently, the worst thing that you can do is go on a "diet". The vast majority of people who follow a "diet" inevitably end up increasing their weight in the long term. This is because the majority of diets that work in the short term aren't sufficiently balanced diets and if you were to follow them for a long time you will very likely end up suffering from malnutrition. Short term diets will enable you to lose weight quickly but these diets cannot be sustained. Sooner or later you will revert to your old eating habits and very likely end up weighing more than you did when you started the diet. Short term diets do work – in the short term; but they should not be considered as a long-term solution to your weight aspirations. Following short-term diets is also called "Yo-yo" dieting and may be harmful to your health.

The reason why there are so many diets on the market is that their creators know that there is an endless stream of dieters who will try their diets and lose weight in the short term. Very few, if any, of these diet creators will claim that their particular diet will cause you to lose the weight that you want to lose and maintain that new weight for the rest of your life. Nobody can eat only grapefruit of grapes or any other single food for the rest of his or her life. You also cannot sustain a greatly reduced food intake for the rest of your life. Excluding certain foods such as pastas, desserts and red meats creates a flawed eating program. And following a particular short term diet periodically for the rest of your life can be detrimental to your health.

It's therefore important to establish exactly what you want to achieve as far as the controlling of your weight is concerned. If you only want to reduce your weight without any thought as to doing this permanently then a "diet" is all you need. But if you want to maintain the weight that you are seeking for the rest of your life you have to create a balanced eating program that will allow you to do this by becoming an ingrained part of your lifestyle. This can only be done over a long period of time and must become a natural part of your lifestyle.

There aren't any beautiful photographs of food in this booklet. The photographs that are here are practical, just like your eating program should be. Decorating your food with flowers and other colorful things won't help you lose weight permanently. An eating program is a serious undertaking and is focused on the food you need to eat; not pretty pictures.

SHORT TERM WEIGHT REDUCTION

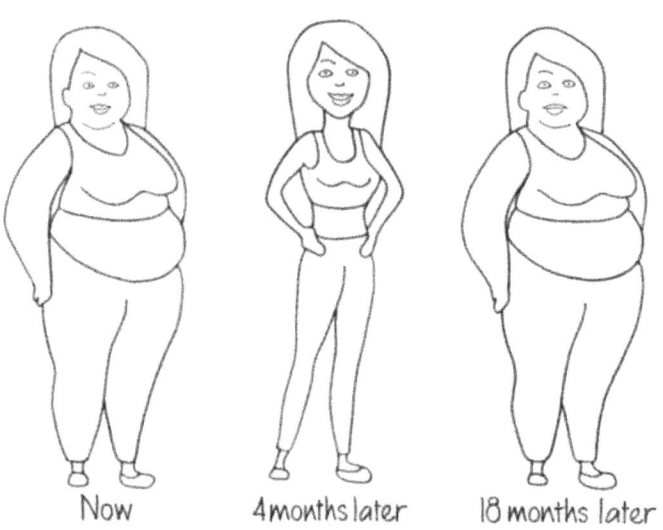

Now   4 months later   18 months later

LONG TERM WEIGHT REDUCTION

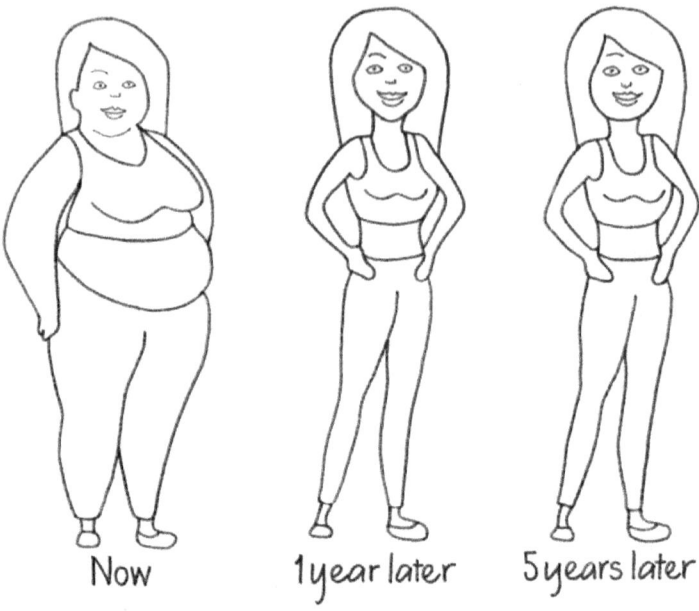

Now   1 year later   5 years later

Creating a long-term eating program takes time and perseverance mainly because it's something that you're going to use for the rest of your life. The ingredients of your program need to be flexible and have as many variations as possible so that they don't become boring. An eating program with its variations needs to be something that you would be comfortable following for the rest of your life. Don't look at an eating program as a short term plan. Imagine yourself following the plan day in and day out for the rest of your life. If you feel comfortable that you can do this then use it. It's not a good idea to keep changing your eating program. This can easily lead to you losing interest in achieving your goal and eventually abandoning the project. Rather keep looking for variations to your original program.

Your eating program has to become a habit and habits don't form overnight. If you are overweight it's usually the result of bad eating habits and a sedentary existence that have become a part of your lifestyle over a lengthy period of time. One of the biggest culprits here is the snacks that you have between meals. To change these habits requires a substantial amount of time and sustained perseverance; also known as **will power**.

If you really want to shock yourself, set aside a small bowl, and each time you add sugar to your food or drink, place a similar amount in the bowl. Do the same with any snacks such as biscuits and sweets/candy. At the end of the day, you'll undoubtedly be shocked at how much sugar is in the bowl and how many biscuits and sweets/candy there are in your collection.

But it's important to understand that changing your eating habits has to be done gradually using a series of small goals that will eventually culminate in you reaching a satisfactory program and your required weight. Rushing a weight reduction program is, in fact, a diet and will inevitably end in failure. Like anything that is worthwhile, changing to a sustainable eating program takes time, patience and considerable discipline. However, it doesn't have to be rigidly adhered to and a certain amount of lenience can, and should be, tolerated.

Adhering to an eating program too rigidly can lead to frustration and unhappiness and result in the plan eventually being abandoned. This is the biggest danger facing someone embarking on a long-term eating program. If the program doesn't become a habit your efforts will be futile. Small digressions, as long as they are recognized as such, can increase your determination to succeed and help you sustain your perseverance. But they must be recognized as temporary digressions and treated as such.

***

So, what is a balanced eating program? A balanced eating program is a plan that lists the types of food and drink that will lead to a reduction in your weight to a healthy level, their combinations, when they should be eaten and, to a certain extent, in what quantities. As an adult, it's your responsibility to be honest with yourself and restrain your urge to eat too large helpings. Your conscience is a good regulator; listen to it.

However, the purpose of this booklet is to give you advice on how to adhere to your eating program and not the quantities that your plan should consist of. Suffice to say that in most cases an effective eating program can be devised using common sense; plenty of fresh fruit and vegetables, limited red meat and a limited consumption of alcohol. Salads, homemade muesli, white meat such as chicken breasts and lean pork, fish, raw nuts, whole-wheat low GI breads, limited sugar and salt and an avoidance of junk food will all contribute to a healthy eating program that will reduce your weight safely, consistently and permanently.

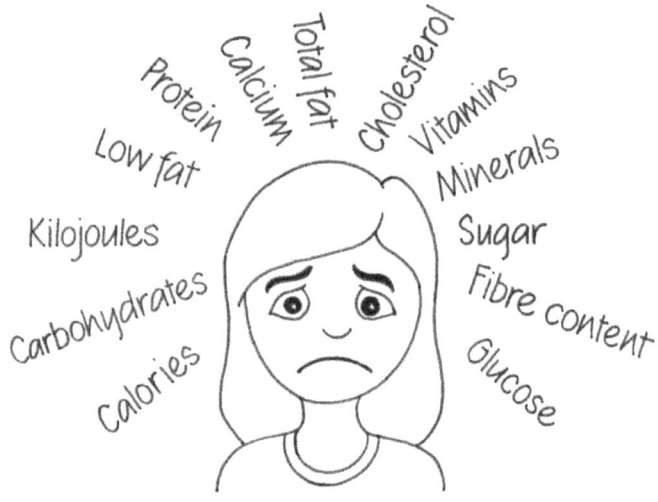

Like so much else in Life, it is best to keep your eating program simple and not be too concerned about kilojoules, fat contents, daily intakes, vitamins and minerals, carbohydrates, protein, nutritional tables and all the other jargon that goes with dieting. Use your common sense and trust in it. Never forget that a healthy eating program will ensure a better quality of life as you grow older.

Don't avoid the advice of nutritionists though. They know what they're talking about and their advice can be and is, very helpful. But again, don't let your eating program become too complicated. Common sense will always prevail. The more complicated you make anything, the more difficult it becomes to master. Keep your program simple, easy to understand and easy to implement and if you feel that it needs refinements then make them. Constantly looking to refine your program will increase you enthusiasm and interest in what you're doing and eating.

Another way of encouraging yourself and building enthusiasm is to follow a particular eating style. Many of the Mediterranean styles such as the Greek and Portuguese styles incorporate many of the ingredients mentioned above as does the Japanese style. Proof that these styles are healthy can be found in the longevity of the citizens of these countries and it can add fun to your program by emulating a foreign style.

The most important thing about an eating program, other than its contents, is time. The longer your eating program takes to become a habit and the more involved you become in it, the more permanent it will be. It's vital to be patient and persevere, regardless of how little progress you believe you are making. Losing half a kilogram in a month might seem discouraging but it's progress and that's what perseverance and success are all about. What it will also tell you, is that your program is slowly becoming a habit and the stronger that habit becomes, the more likely it is to become permanent. Set your target weight but never your target date.

***

There are a number of things that you can do to maintain your progress and finally achieve the weight that you are aiming for permanently.

1. Don't procrastinate when presented with a food temptation. Be strong, say "no" to yourself and walk away quickly. The longer you contemplate purchasing the tempting item, the more likely you are to break your resolution and make the purchase.

2. Where possible, avoid bakeries and bakery departments that offer aromatic food. Many of these entities actually have artificial aromas to entice people to buy their products.

3. Don't buy on impulse. Make a list of what food products you need before leaving to do your shopping and stick to it. Statistics show that 30% of all purchases made in supermarkets are impulse purchases. Congratulate and reward yourself each time you arrive home without having made an impulse purchase.

4. Make out your shopping list after having a meal. This will eliminate the temptation of listing unnecessary food products because you are hungry.

5. Do your shopping as soon after you've had a meal as you can as this will also eliminate the temptation to buy unnecessary food products simply because you're hungry. You also won't be quite so ready to taste food samples offered by sales people.

6. Take pride in resisting temptation and reward yourself when you overcome a temptation. The more you do this the easier it will be the next time you're faced with a difficult temptation.

7. Create a mental picture of what you'll look like in five or ten years time if you continue with your eating program. This is a great way to keep yourself out of temptation's way and strengthen your resolve to succeed. The more vivid your picture is the more of a positive effect it will have. Also bear in mind that your subconscious mind, the mind that affects you body, will be influenced by your mental image and influence your resolve positively. Mental images have amazing power.

8. Tell your friends about your progress. This will demonstrate and strengthen your commitment. Many people hope that others will fail so as to boost their own inability to do what you're doing. See and enjoy their surprise and envy when you finally succeed.

9. In the beginning strive to maintain a steady but small weight loss consistently as this is an indication that you are on the road to success. Don't be disappointed if your progress is interrupted by a small weight gain. Study your recent endeavors and try to see what has caused this problem. Usually, in hindsight, this is very obvious, but make sure that you learn from the fault so that it doesn't crop up again. Small failures are important as long as you learn from them and adjust your plan accordingly. The longer it takes you to reach your weight goal the more likely it is that it will become a permanent part of your life once you reach that goal.

10. The best exercise that you can do while implementing your eating and weight reduction program is shaking your head and saying "No".

***

Spend a lot of time establishing your eating program but remember that it can be changed or refined if it doesn't meet your expectations or becomes boring. Get as much advice as possible but try to keep your plan as simple as possible. Remember that this plan will have a lasting effect on your life and needs to be easy to follow. As you progress, try to avoid adding unnecessary details as these can cause you to lose sight of your ultimate goal and get engrossed in distracting unimportant detail.

Create your mental image as early as possible as this is a very important part of sustaining your momentum. The more vivid your mental image is, the more effective it will be. Remember that a small series of progressive weight losses is far more important than one large weight reduction. In fact, try to avoid large weight reductions as they will weaken your cause and can easily lead to disappointment when they are not sustained.

Achieving a lifestyle that enables you to maintain a healthy weight permanently is a wonderful achievement and something that you will cherish and never regret.

SUGGESTED EATING PROGRAM

BREAKFAST

Monday-Friday: homemade muesli – 5 tablespoons of rolled oats, half a teaspoon of brown sugar, 1 dessertspoon of raisins or sultanas, 1 dessertspoon of raw nuts, 1 chopped-up apple, 1 sliced banana, low fat milk. There are plenty of fruit variations that you can use.

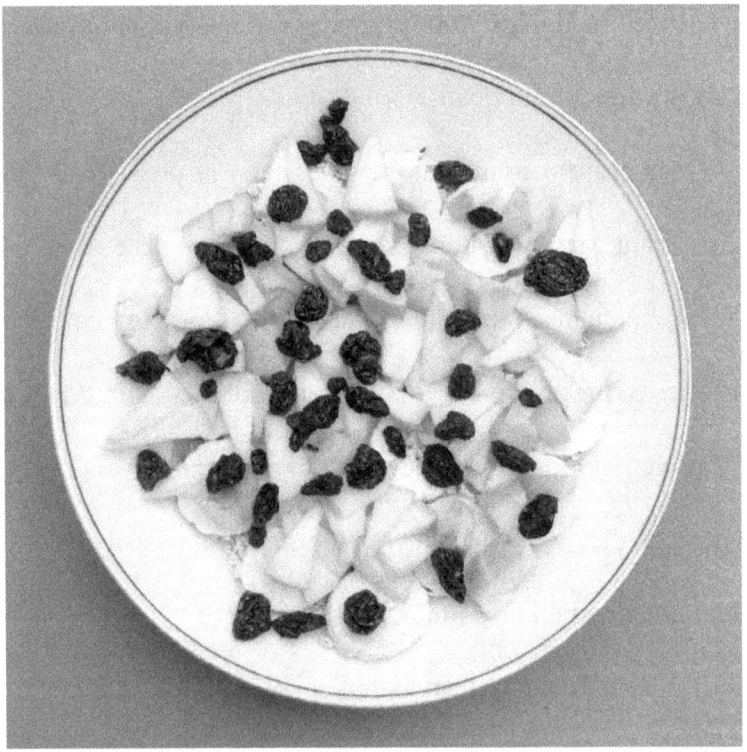

Rolled oats, sugar, raw peanuts, banana, apple, raisins and low fat milk

***

Saturday: cooked oats porridge – 5 tablespoons of raw rolled oats, half a teaspoon of brown sugar, low fat milk OR sorghum porridge OR 4 scrambled/poached eggs on 2 slices of whole wheat toast.

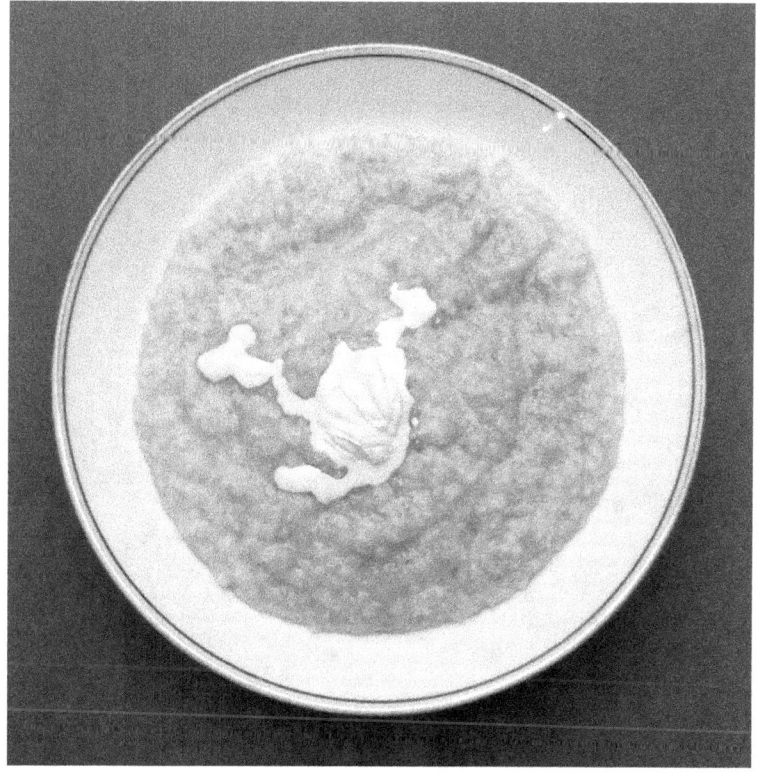

Rolled oats, sugar, canola margarine and low fat milk

***

Sunday: tomato and onion mix – 3 large tomatoes, 1 chopped-up onion, canola oil/olive oil, spices/herbs, 1 slice whole wheat bread, 1 banana, 3 scrambled/poached eggs.

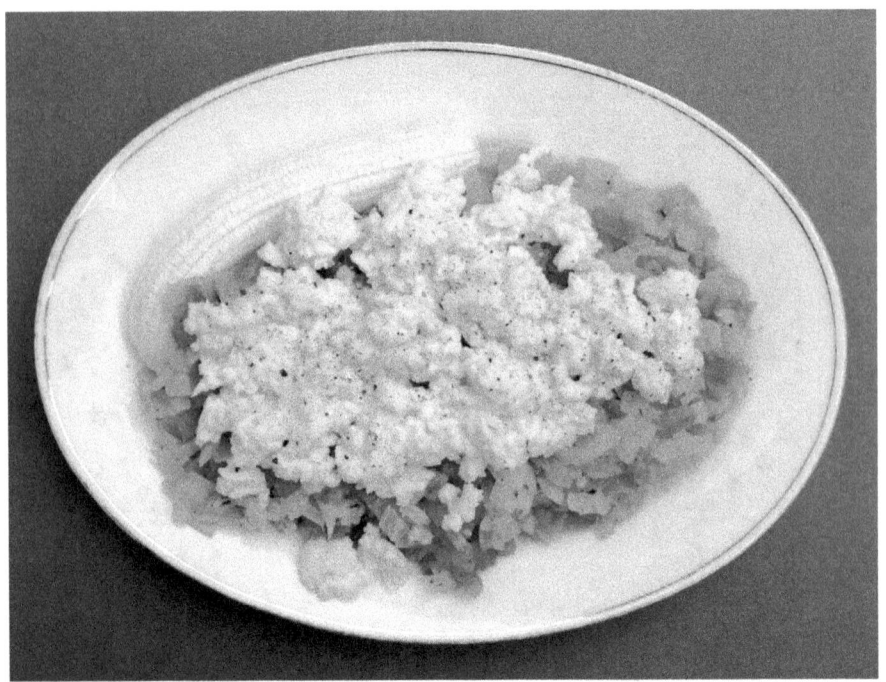

Tomato, onion, banana and scrambled eggs

***

LUNCH

Monday-Saturday: 2 whole wheat sandwiches with canola margarine, sliced apple/banana/tomato and canola mayonnaise OR peanut butter OR tuna and canola mayonnaise filling and a salad.

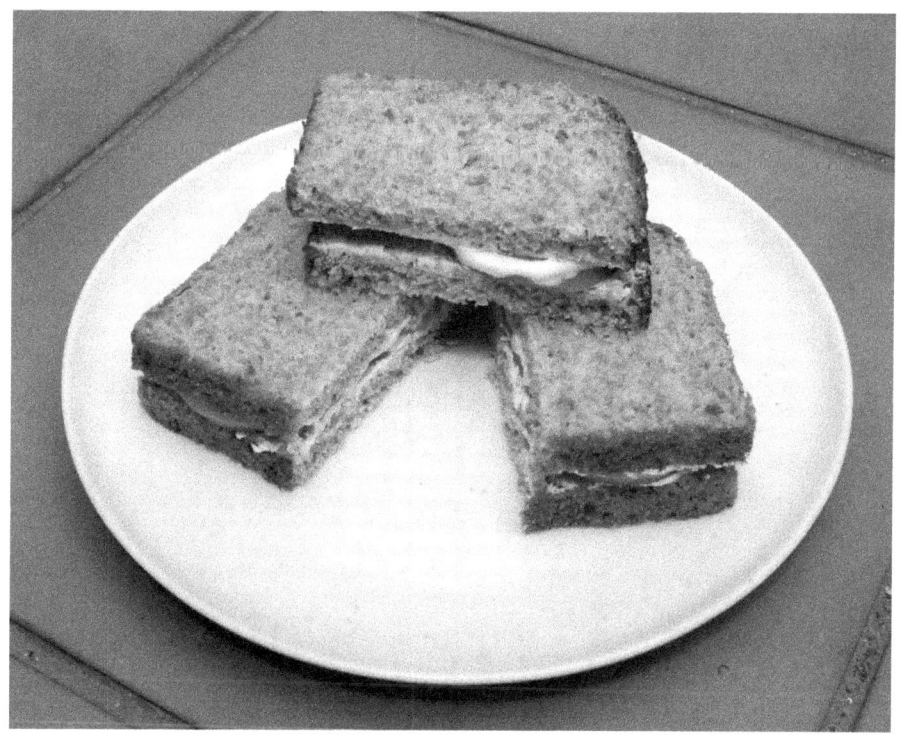

Low GI brown bread, canola margarine, tomato and canola mayonnaise

OR

Soup and 3 slices of whole wheat brown bread with a salad of your choice.

***

Sunday: boiled/grilled vegetables, 1 banana, 1 skinless chicken fillet/pork neck steak or fish and a salad of your choice.

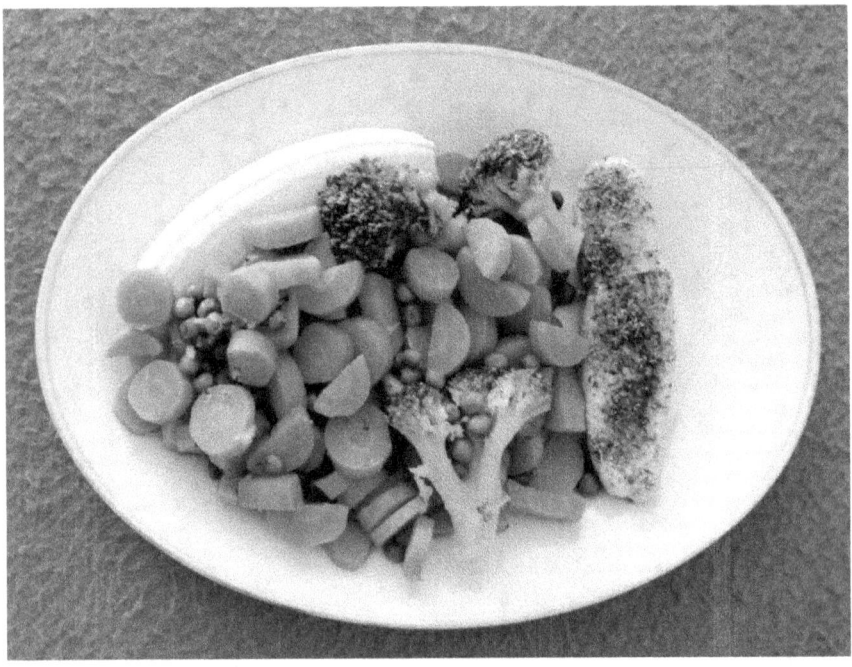

Skinless chicken breast, mixed herbs, carrots, broccoli, peas and banana

***

SUPPER

Monday-Wednesday: boiled/grilled vegetables, 1 banana, 1 piece middle cut mackerel/skinless chicken breast/pork neck steak and a salad.

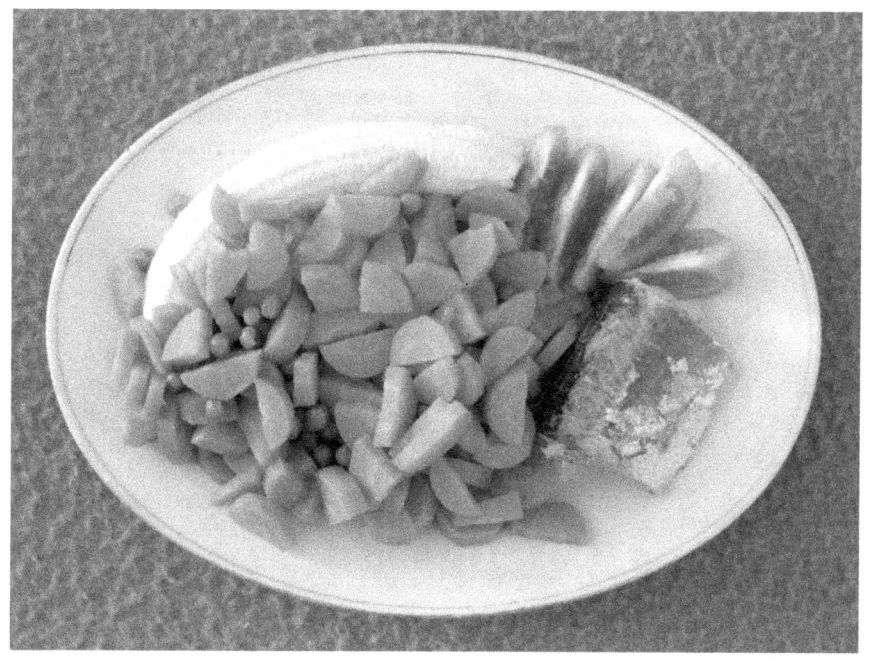

Middle cut mackerel, carrots, peas, tomato and banana

***

Thursday: 2 dessertspoons barley and 2 dessertspoons brown rice OR a handful of spaghetti with mashed middle cut mackerel or tuna and canola mayonnaise and a salad.

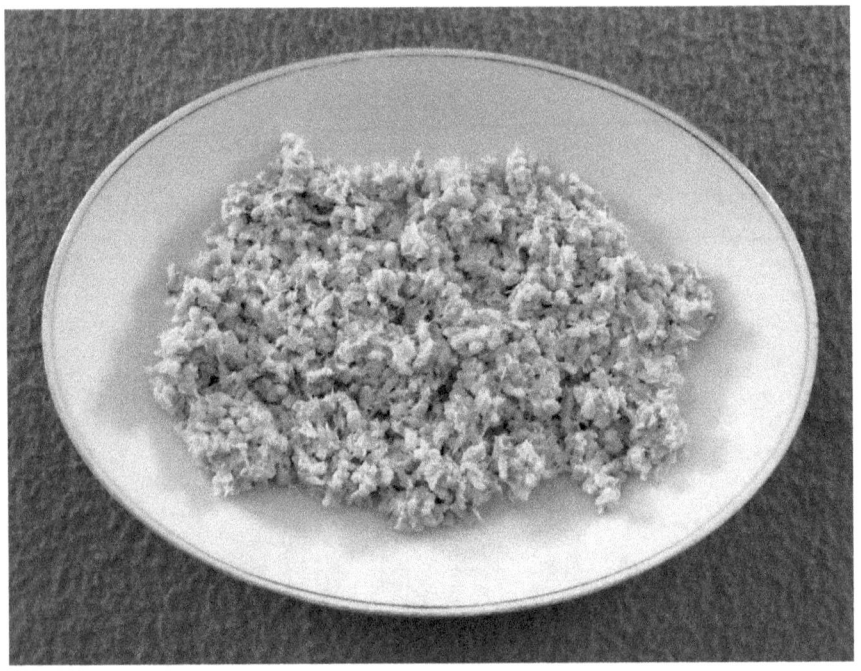

Brown rice, barley, middle cut mackerel and mayonnaise

***

Friday-Saturday: 2 dessertspoons barley and 2 dessertspoons brown rice OR a handful of spaghetti with soya mince and bean topping* and a salad.

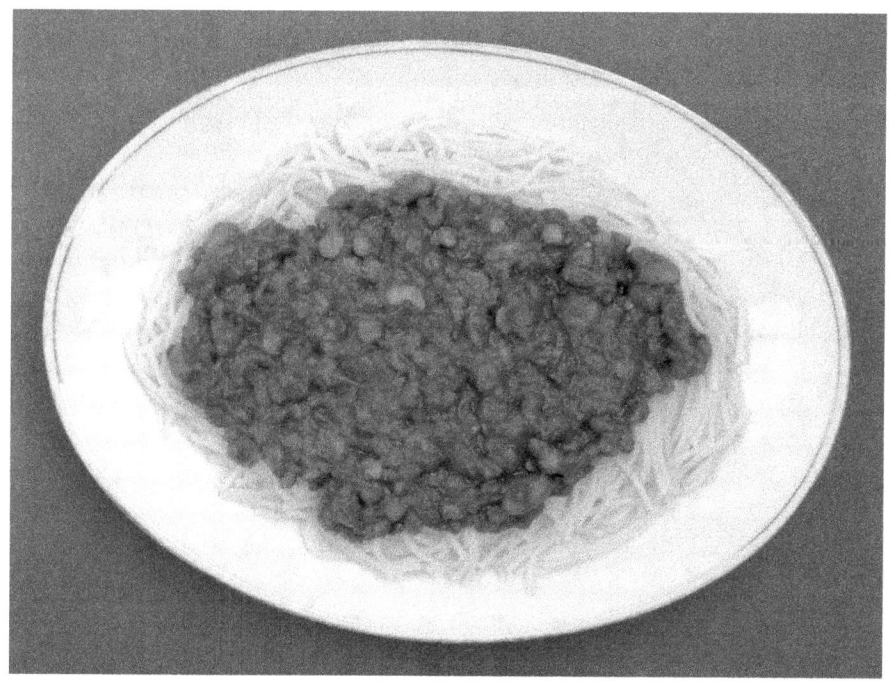

Spaghetti and soya mince and bean topping*

Sunday: 4 poached eggs on 2 slices of toasted whole wheat bread

***

All the above meals, except the breakfasts, can and should be augmented with a fresh green salad. You can never eat too much salad; just ease up on the salad dressings.

*SOYA MINCE AND BEAN TOPPING (serves six)

Ingredients: 500 grams (20 ounces) soya mince, ½ can tomato pure, 150 grams (6 ounces) red beans, 150 grams (6 ounces) white beans, 150 grams (6 ounces) split peas, 1 chopped onion, 1 packet beef soup powder, herbs and spices

Method: cook the beans and split peas until soft, cook soya mince, chopped onion and spices to taste and mix with beans.

SNACKS: raw peanuts, raw carrots, biscuits (1 small packet a week), chocolate (2 X 80 gram (3 ounces) slabs a week)

LIQUIDS: tea, coffee, lemonade made from lemon juice, a little sugar and water, wine (1-2 glasses a day)

By following this program and its variations, you will never increase your weight even if you break away from it over weekends by enjoying a family Sunday roast with plenty of vegetables, a sweet and a few glasses of wine or an evening at a restaurant with a juicy steak, vegetables, fries and a few beers followed by a sweet and coffee. By the following Wednesday you'll be back to your normal weight.

Achieving a permanent eating program that guarantees a lifestyle free from continual temporary weight reduction stints requires self control and perseverance but whatever sacrifice this necessitates will pale into insignificance compared to the enjoyable weight stabilization and good health that you will experience.

www.ingramcontent.com/pod-product-compliance
Lightning Source LLC
Chambersburg PA
CBHW072017280526
45788CB00005B/2077